I0774579

LIVER DISEASE GUIDE

Journey to Optimal Liver Wellness

BY

Dr. Luna Jefferson

Copyright

No part of this book should be copied, reproduced without the author's permission © 2023

TABLE OF CONTENT

INTRODUCTION

Welcome to the exploration of a vital organ that plays a silent yet profound role in our well-being—the liver. This book is an insightful journey into the intricate world of liver diseases, tailored for those seeking knowledge, prevention, or guidance through the challenges of living with such conditions.

In the opening chapters, we unveil the liver's complexity, unraveling its anatomical wonders and multifaceted functions. As the cornerstone of our body's metabolic processes, the liver deserves our attention and understanding. We delve into the prevalence of liver diseases globally, emphasizing the importance of awareness and preventative measures.

The subsequent chapters bridge the knowledge gap, detailing various types of liver diseases, from the well-known hepatitis variants to the insidious non-alcoholic fatty liver disease and cirrhosis. We explore the risk factors contributing to these conditions, empowering readers with practical steps to safeguard their liver health.

This book is a beacon for those navigating a new diagnosis or seeking comprehensive insights into liver diseases they've battled for years. From symptoms and early detection to diagnostic tools and treatment options, each page is a guide, providing clarity and support. As we journey together, let us unlock the doors to understanding, prevention, and holistic well-being in the realm of liver health.

Brief overview of the liver's functions and importance for overall health.

The liver, a marvel of biological engineering, is a dynamic organ with a repertoire of vital functions crucial for sustaining our overall health. Nestled beneath the ribcage, this organ acts as the body's metabolic hub, orchestrating processes essential for life. One of its primary roles is detoxification, filtering and neutralizing toxins from the bloodstream. As a metabolic powerhouse, the liver processes nutrients, converting food into energy and synthesizing proteins critical for bodily functions.

Crucially, the liver regulates glucose levels, ensuring a steady energy supply for the body. It also stores essential vitamins and minerals, releasing them when needed. Blood clotting factors, vital for wound healing, are synthesized in the liver, underlining its indispensable role in our defense against injuries. Furthermore, the liver produces bile, aiding in the digestion and absorption of fats.

The importance of the liver reverberates throughout the body, impacting various systems and contributing to overall well-being. Any disruption to these intricate processes can lead to a cascade of health issues. Understanding the significance of the liver's functions is fundamental to appreciating its role in maintaining balance and harmony within the body, underscoring the necessity of its optimal health for our overall well-being.

The prevalence of liver diseases globally and the impact on public health.

Liver diseases cast a pervasive shadow on global public health, with a prevalence that spans continents and communities. The World Health Organization estimates that millions of individuals worldwide are affected by various forms of liver disorders, creating a substantial burden on healthcare systems and societies. Hepatitis viruses, in particular, contribute significantly to this global health challenge, with millions of new infections reported annually.

The impact of liver diseases on public health is multifaceted. Beyond the immediate toll on individuals' well-being, these conditions strain healthcare resources, demanding extensive medical interventions, from diagnostic tests to advanced treatments. Chronic liver diseases, such as cirrhosis, escalate the burden further, often requiring long-term management and, in severe cases, liver transplantation.

Furthermore, the economic implications are substantial, encompassing healthcare costs, lost productivity, and the societal toll of lives disrupted by illness. The global nature of liver diseases underscores the need for concerted efforts in prevention, early detection, and accessible treatment options. Public health initiatives, vaccination campaigns, and awareness programs play a pivotal role in mitigating the prevalence and impact of liver diseases, offering a glimmer of hope in the pursuit of a healthier world.

CHAPTER ONE

Understanding the Liver

Understanding the liver goes beyond recognizing it as a vital organ; it involves unraveling the intricacies of its structure and functions that are fundamental to human physiology. Anatomically, the liver is a large, reddish-brown organ situated in the upper right side of the abdomen, protected by the ribcage. Comprising two main lobes, it is intricately connected to the circulatory and digestive systems.

The liver's functions are as diverse as they are critical. Acting as the body's metabolic powerhouse, it processes nutrients from the bloodstream, converting them into energy and synthesizing essential proteins. Detoxification is a key role, as the liver filters toxins, drugs, and other harmful substances, safeguarding the body from potential damage.

Moreover, the liver regulates blood glucose levels, stores vitamins and minerals, and produces bile—a substance crucial for digesting fats. Its role in synthesizing clotting factors contributes to wound healing and ensures the body's defense against bleeding.

Understanding the liver lays the foundation for comprehending the impact of liver diseases and appreciating the significance of maintaining its optimal health. It serves as a sentinel, tirelessly working to sustain the delicate balance necessary for the body's overall well-being and functionality.

Anatomy and structure of the liver

The liver, an organ of remarkable complexity, boasts an intricate anatomy finely tuned to execute its myriad functions. Positioned in the upper right quadrant of the abdomen, beneath the ribcage, the liver is a wedge-shaped organ divided into two main lobes—right and left—each further subdivided into lobules. These lobules house thousands of hepatic cells, the liver's functional units.

A network of blood vessels intricately weaves through the liver, with the hepatic artery supplying oxygen-rich blood and the portal vein delivering nutrient-rich blood from the digestive system. This dual blood supply is crucial for the liver's metabolic functions, as it processes nutrients, detoxifies harmful substances, and regulates glucose levels.

The liver's structural brilliance extends to its biliary system, which includes bile ducts that transport bile, a digestive fluid produced by the liver, to the gallbladder for storage and subsequent release into the small intestine. Bile plays a pivotal role in breaking down fats for absorption.

Microscopically, hepatic cells, or hepatocytes, form the liver's parenchyma, where metabolic processes unfold. Understanding the intricacies of the liver's anatomy unveils the foundation for comprehending its diverse functions, emphasizing the organ's pivotal role in maintaining homeostasis within the human body.

Functions of the liver, including detoxification, metabolism, and synthesis of proteins.

The liver stands as a metabolic maestro, orchestrating an array of functions vital for sustaining life. One of its key roles is detoxification, where it acts as a sophisticated filter, removing toxins, drugs, and harmful substances from the bloodstream. Through intricate enzymatic processes, the liver transforms these potentially dangerous compounds into water-soluble substances that can be excreted from the body.

Metabolism is another cornerstone of the liver's functions. It processes nutrients absorbed from the digestive tract, regulating glucose levels, and storing excess glucose in the form of glycogen. In times of need, the liver converts glycogen back into glucose, ensuring a steady supply of energy for the body.

The synthesis of proteins is a paramount responsibility of the liver. It produces a myriad of proteins, including albumin, essential for maintaining blood volume and pressure, and clotting factors crucial for coagulation and wound healing. Additionally, the liver synthesizes proteins involved in immune function, contributing to the body's defense mechanisms.

Understanding these multifaceted functions emphasizes the liver's indispensable role in maintaining physiological balance. Its capacity for detoxification, metabolic regulation, and protein synthesis underscores the intricate and integral nature of this organ in supporting overall health and well-being.

CHAPTER TWO

Common Types of Liver Diseases

Liver diseases encompass a spectrum of conditions that can impact the organ's structure and function, posing significant health challenges. Among the most prevalent are hepatitis infections, classified as A, B, C, D, and E. These viral infections can lead to inflammation of the liver, with chronic cases potentially progressing to cirrhosis.

Liver diseases manifest in various forms, each with distinct features and presentations. Understanding these common types is crucial for early detection and effective management. Here are some prevalent liver diseases:

1. Hepatitis:
   - **Features:** Hepatitis is inflammation of the liver, often caused by viral infections (A, B, C, D, and E). Symptoms

may include fatigue, jaundice, abdominal pain, nausea, and vomiting.

   - **Presentation:** Hepatitis A and E typically result from contaminated food or water, while B, C, and D spread through blood and bodily fluids. Chronic hepatitis can lead to cirrhosis.

2. Cirrhosis:

   - **Features:** Cirrhosis is late-stage scarring of the liver tissue, often a result of long-term liver damage. Symptoms include fatigue, weakness, easy bruising, swelling in the legs, and confusion.

   - **Presentation:** Cirrhosis can develop from various liver diseases, including chronic hepatitis and alcohol-related liver disease. It progresses slowly, and symptoms may not appear until significant damage has occurred.

3. Non-alcoholic Fatty Liver Disease (NAFLD):

   - **Features:** NAFLD involves the accumulation of fat in the liver, unrelated to alcohol consumption. It ranges from simple fatty liver to non-alcoholic steatohepatitis (NASH), which can lead to cirrhosis.

   - **Presentation:** Often asymptomatic in the early stages, symptoms may include fatigue, abdominal discomfort, and weight loss as the disease progresses.

4. Alcoholic Liver Disease:

- **Features:** Caused by excessive alcohol consumption over time, alcoholic liver disease encompasses fatty liver, alcoholic hepatitis, and cirrhosis.
- **Presentation:** Early stages may be asymptomatic or present with vague symptoms. Alcoholic hepatitis can cause jaundice, abdominal pain, and liver failure, while cirrhosis manifests with advanced symptoms.

5. Liver Cancer:
- **Features:** Primary liver cancer originates in the liver, while secondary liver cancer spreads from other organs.
- **Presentation:** Symptoms include unexplained weight loss, abdominal pain, jaundice, and swelling. Early stages may be asymptomatic.

6. Autoimmune Hepatitis:
- **Features:** An immune system malfunction where the body attacks liver cells, leading to inflammation.
- **Presentation:** Symptoms include fatigue, joint pain, abdominal discomfort, and jaundice. It may progress to cirrhosis if left untreated.

Understanding the distinct features and presentations of these common liver diseases is crucial for timely diagnosis and appropriate medical intervention. Early detection improves the prognosis and allows for effective management strategies. Individuals experiencing symptoms or at risk should seek prompt medical attention for a comprehensive evaluation.

Hepatitis (A, B, C, D, E): Causes, symptoms, and prevention.

Hepatitis, a group of viral infections affecting the liver, comprises various strains denoted by letters A, B, C, D, and E, each with its distinct characteristics. Hepatitis A typically spreads through contaminated food or water, causing acute infection. Symptoms include fever, fatigue, and jaundice. Vaccination and practicing good hygiene are effective preventive measures.

Hepatitis B is transmitted through infected blood and bodily fluids. It can lead to chronic infection, cirrhosis, and liver cancer. Symptoms range from mild to severe, and prevention involves vaccination, safe sex practices, and avoiding shared needles.

Hepatitis C is primarily spread through contact with infected blood and can become chronic, leading to cirrhosis and liver cancer. It often presents with mild or no symptoms initially. Prevention involves avoiding exposure to infected blood and, for those at risk, regular testing.

Hepatitis D is a unique virus that only infects those already infected with hepatitis B. It can exacerbate the severity of hepatitis B. Preventing hepatitis D involves preventing hepatitis B through vaccination.

Hepatitis E is typically transmitted through contaminated water and resembles hepatitis A. It is usually acute, with symptoms including jaundice and fatigue. Prevention involves safe drinking water practices and proper sanitation.

Understanding the causes, symptoms, and preventive measures for each hepatitis strain is critical in controlling the spread of these infections and reducing their impact on liver health. Vaccination stands out as a key strategy in preventing several forms of hepatitis, underlining the importance of global immunization efforts.

Cirrhosis: Causes, progression, and complications.

Cirrhosis stands as a progressive and irreversible scarring of the liver tissue, often emerging as a consequence of chronic liver diseases such as hepatitis and long-term alcohol abuse. The liver, normally a regenerative organ, attempts to repair itself when injured. However, in the face of persistent damage, the healing process leads to the accumulation of scar tissue, disrupting the liver's structure and impeding its vital functions.

The causes of cirrhosis are diverse, with chronic viral infections, especially hepatitis B and C, alcohol-related liver disease, non-alcoholic fatty liver disease (NAFLD), and autoimmune hepatitis being common culprits. As cirrhosis advances, the liver's ability to perform essential tasks like detoxification, synthesis of proteins, and regulation of blood flow diminishes.

The progression of cirrhosis unfolds in stages, with early symptoms often subtle or absent. Over time, individuals may experience fatigue, weakness, abdominal pain, and fluid retention. As cirrhosis advances, complications arise, including portal hypertension, which can lead to the development of varices (enlarged blood vessels) and increased risk of bleeding. Additionally, impaired liver function can result in hepatic encephalopathy, a condition affecting cognitive function.

Understanding the causes, recognizing early symptoms, and addressing underlying liver conditions are critical in managing cirrhosis. Lifestyle changes, medications, and, in severe cases, liver transplantation may be necessary to alleviate the impact of this progressive liver disease.

Non-alcoholic Fatty Liver Disease (NAFLD) and alcoholic liver disease

Non-alcoholic Fatty Liver Disease (NAFLD) and Alcoholic Liver Disease (ALD) are two distinct yet interconnected liver conditions, both posing significant health concerns.

NAFLD is characterized by the accumulation of fat in liver cells, not caused by excessive alcohol consumption. It is often associated with obesity, insulin resistance, and metabolic syndrome. NAFLD exists on a spectrum, ranging from simple steatosis (fat buildup) to non-alcoholic steatohepatitis (NASH), which involves inflammation and liver cell damage. Over time, NAFLD can progress to cirrhosis and increase the risk of liver cancer. Lifestyle changes, including a balanced diet and regular exercise, form the cornerstone of NAFLD management.

Conversely, ALD results from prolonged and excessive alcohol consumption, leading to liver inflammation, fatty liver, alcoholic hepatitis, and ultimately cirrhosis. Genetic factors also play a role in susceptibility to ALD. Reducing or eliminating alcohol intake is crucial in managing ALD, and support from healthcare professionals or support groups may be beneficial.

While NAFLD and ALD have distinct triggers, both underscore the liver's vulnerability to metabolic imbalances. Understanding the contributing factors, adopting healthy lifestyles, and seeking timely medical intervention are pivotal in managing these liver conditions and preserving overall health.

CHAPTER THREE

Risk Factors and Prevention

Risk factors for liver diseases span a spectrum of lifestyle choices, genetic predispositions, and environmental influences. Understanding and mitigating these factors are pivotal in preventing the onset and progression of various liver conditions.

1. Unhealthy Diet: Diets high in saturated fats, sugars, and processed foods contribute to obesity and non-alcoholic fatty liver disease (NAFLD). A balanced diet with an emphasis on fruits, vegetables, and whole grains is crucial for liver health.

2. Excessive Alcohol Consumption: Chronic and heavy alcohol consumption is a significant risk factor for alcoholic liver disease. Moderation or abstinence from alcohol is key in preventing alcohol-related liver damage.

3. Viral Infections: Hepatitis viruses (B and C, in particular) are major contributors to liver diseases. Vaccination, safe sex practices, and avoiding sharing needles are effective preventive measures.

4. Genetic Factors: Some liver diseases, such as hemochromatosis and Wilson's disease, have a genetic component. Understanding family medical history and seeking genetic counseling can help manage these risks.

5. Obesity and Metabolic Syndrome: Being overweight or obese increases the likelihood of developing NAFLD and other metabolic disorders. Maintaining a healthy weight through regular exercise and a balanced diet is crucial.

Preventive measures involve lifestyle modifications, vaccination, and regular health check-ups. Public health initiatives promoting awareness and education about liver health, along with accessible healthcare resources, are essential components of a comprehensive approach to prevent liver diseases on both individual and societal levels.

Lifestyle factors contributing to liver disease

Lifestyle factors play a pivotal role in the development and progression of liver diseases, emphasizing the profound impact of daily choices on the health of this vital organ.

1. Diet: High intake of saturated fats, sugars, and processed foods can lead to obesity and insulin resistance, contributing to the development of non-alcoholic fatty liver disease (NAFLD). A diet rich in fruits, vegetables, and whole grains supports liver health by providing essential nutrients and promoting a healthy weight.

2. Alcohol Consumption: Excessive and prolonged alcohol intake is a well-established risk factor for liver diseases, including alcoholic liver disease. Chronic alcohol abuse can lead to inflammation, fatty liver, alcoholic hepatitis, and cirrhosis. Moderating alcohol consumption or abstaining is crucial for liver health.

3. Sedentary Lifestyle: Lack of physical activity is associated with obesity and metabolic syndrome, both linked to liver diseases. Regular exercise promotes weight management, improves insulin sensitivity, and contributes to overall liver function.

4. Smoking: Smoking has been identified as a risk factor for liver diseases, including liver cancer. The harmful substances in tobacco smoke can exacerbate liver damage and hinder the organ's ability to regenerate.

5. Poor Hydration: Inadequate water intake can affect liver function, as water is essential for detoxification processes. Staying well-hydrated supports the liver in effectively eliminating toxins from the body.

Making conscious choices in these areas—adopting a balanced diet, moderating alcohol intake, staying physically active, quitting smoking, and maintaining proper hydration—can significantly reduce the risk of liver diseases and contribute to overall well-being.

Importance of vaccinations for hepatitis.

Vaccinations for hepatitis stand as a critical pillar in public health, playing a pivotal role in preventing the spread of this viral infection and mitigating the associated risks to liver health. Hepatitis viruses, especially types B and A, can lead to severe liver diseases, including chronic infections, cirrhosis, and liver cancer. Vaccination against these viruses has proven to be highly effective in averting these potentially life-threatening consequences.

Hepatitis B vaccination, administered in a series of shots, is a routine immunization recommended for infants, adolescents, and adults, particularly those at higher risk due to medical conditions, occupation, or lifestyle choices. By stimulating the immune system to produce antibodies against the virus, the vaccine provides robust protection.

Hepatitis A vaccination is another crucial preventive measure, safeguarding individuals from the acute infection caused by consuming contaminated food or water. This vaccine is recommended for travelers to areas with high hepatitis A prevalence and for certain at-risk populations.

The importance of these vaccinations extends beyond individual health, contributing to the broader goal of public health by reducing the incidence of hepatitis-related liver diseases and lessening the burden on healthcare systems. Emphasizing the significance of timely vaccinations underscores their role as a cornerstone in the collective effort to promote liver health and prevent the spread of hepatitis.

Tips for maintaining a healthy liver through diet and exercise.

Maintaining a healthy liver is closely linked to lifestyle choices, with a focus on diet and exercise playing a paramount role in supporting optimal liver function. Here are key tips to promote liver health through these lifestyle factors:

1. Balanced Diet: Adopting a well-balanced and nutritious diet is fundamental. Include a variety of fruits, vegetables, whole grains, and lean proteins in your meals. These foods provide essential nutrients, antioxidants, and fiber, promoting overall health and supporting the liver's metabolic functions.

2. Moderate Fat Intake: Limit saturated and trans fats in your diet, as excessive fat consumption can contribute to non-alcoholic fatty liver disease (NAFLD). Opt for healthy fats like those found in avocados, nuts, and olive oil.

3. Hydration: Adequate water intake is crucial for liver health. Water supports the liver in detoxification processes, helping flush out toxins and waste products from the body.

4. Limit Alcohol Consumption: If you consume alcohol, do so in moderation. Excessive alcohol intake is a leading cause of liver diseases, including cirrhosis. Guidelines recommend moderate drinking, which is up to one drink per day for women and up to two drinks per day for men.

5. Regular Exercise: Engage in regular physical activity, as exercise contributes to weight management and improves insulin sensitivity. Both are crucial for preventing obesity and metabolic syndrome, which are risk factors for liver diseases.

Incorporating these tips into your lifestyle fosters a holistic approach to liver health, reducing the risk of liver diseases and promoting overall well-being.

CHAPTER FOUR

Symptoms and Early Detection

Symptoms of liver diseases can vary widely, and in many cases, they may not manifest until the condition has advanced. Early detection is crucial for effective intervention and management. Understanding the potential symptoms prompts proactive health-seeking behavior and timely medical evaluation.

Common symptoms of liver diseases include fatigue, weakness, unexplained weight loss, nausea, and abdominal pain. Jaundice, characterized by yellowing of the skin and eyes, often indicates liver dysfunction. Dark urine and pale-colored stools may also be indicative of liver issues.

In the early stages of liver diseases, individuals may experience subtle signs or none at all. Therefore, routine medical check-ups and screenings play a pivotal role in early detection. Blood tests can assess liver function, measuring enzyme levels and detecting markers of liver inflammation. Imaging studies, such as ultrasounds or CT scans, provide visual insights into the liver's condition.

For those at higher risk, such as individuals with a family history of liver diseases or those with chronic viral infections, regular screenings are particularly important. Timely detection allows for early intervention and lifestyle modifications, offering the best chance for effective management and improved outcomes.

Promoting awareness of these symptoms and advocating for routine screenings can empower individuals to take charge of their liver health, facilitating early detection and increasing the likelihood of positive health outcomes.

Common symptoms of liver disease

Common symptoms of liver disease serve as crucial indicators that prompt individuals to seek medical attention for a thorough evaluation of their liver health. While symptoms can vary depending on the specific liver condition, some common manifestations include:

1. Fatigue: Persistent tiredness and weakness are prevalent in liver diseases due to the organ's compromised ability to store and release energy.

2. Jaundice: Yellowing of the skin and eyes is a classic sign of liver dysfunction, indicating a buildup of bilirubin, a yellow pigment.

3. Abdominal Pain: Discomfort or pain in the upper right abdomen may be indicative of liver inflammation or enlargement.

4. Unexplained Weight Loss: Sudden and unexplained weight loss can occur as the liver struggles to perform its metabolic functions efficiently.

5. Nausea and Vomiting: Digestive issues, including nausea and vomiting, are common in liver diseases, disrupting the normal processing of nutrients.

6. Changes in Urine and Stool Color: Dark urine and pale-colored stools may signal liver problems, reflecting disruptions in the bile production and excretion processes.

7. Swelling: Fluid retention, leading to swelling in the abdomen (ascites) or legs, is a consequence of impaired liver function and blood flow.

These symptoms underscore the importance of paying attention to one's body and seeking medical advice if any concerning signs arise. Early recognition and diagnosis are critical for effective management and treatment of liver diseases, emphasizing the significance of regular health check-ups and screenings.

The importance of regular check-ups and screenings

Regular check-ups and screenings are instrumental in maintaining overall health and play a pivotal role in the early detection and prevention of various medical conditions, including liver diseases. Here's why these health assessments are crucial:

1. Early Detection: Many health issues, including liver diseases, may not exhibit noticeable symptoms in their early stages. Regular screenings enable healthcare professionals to identify potential problems before symptoms manifest, allowing for timely intervention and treatment.

2. Prevention: Screening tests can detect risk factors or early signs of certain conditions, empowering individuals to make lifestyle changes that can prevent the progression of diseases.

3. Improved Outcomes: Early detection often leads to more effective and less invasive treatment options, resulting in better outcomes for individuals facing health challenges.

4. Disease Management: For chronic conditions like liver diseases, regular check-ups provide an opportunity for healthcare providers to monitor the progression of the disease, adjust treatment plans, and offer guidance on lifestyle modifications.

5. Peace of Mind: Regular check-ups offer reassurance for individuals, fostering a sense of proactive health management and reducing anxiety associated with potential health concerns.

In the context of liver health, routine check-ups may include blood tests to assess liver function, imaging studies to visualize the liver's condition, and screenings for viral infections like hepatitis. The importance of regular health assessments cannot be overstated, as they serve as a cornerstone for preventive healthcare and contribute significantly to maintaining overall well-being.

Diagnostic tests for liver conditions

Diagnostic tests for liver conditions are essential in evaluating the health and functionality of this vital organ. These tests aid healthcare professionals in identifying various liver diseases, assessing their severity, and formulating appropriate treatment plans. Here are key diagnostic tests commonly used for liver conditions:

1. Blood Tests: Liver function tests measure the levels of enzymes, proteins, and other substances in the blood that indicate how well the liver is working. Elevated levels of certain enzymes can suggest liver damage or inflammation.

2. Imaging Studies: Ultrasound, CT scans, and MRI scans provide detailed images of the liver's structure, helping identify abnormalities, such as tumors, cysts, or signs of cirrhosis.

3. FibroScan or Elastography: These non-invasive tests assess liver stiffness, helping determine the degree of fibrosis or scarring. They are valuable in evaluating the progression of liver diseases.

4. Liver Biopsy: In some cases, a small tissue sample is taken from the liver for microscopic examination. This helps diagnose the specific liver condition, assess the extent of damage, and guide treatment decisions.

5. Viral Hepatitis Tests: Specific blood tests can identify the presence of hepatitis viruses (A, B, C, D, or E) and help determine the appropriate course of treatment.

These diagnostic tests are instrumental in providing a comprehensive picture of liver health, allowing for accurate diagnoses and tailored treatment strategies. Early and precise identification of liver conditions through these tests is crucial for effective management and improved patient outcomes.

CHAPTER FIVE

Diagnosis and Medical Evaluation

Diagnosis and medical evaluation are integral steps in understanding and addressing liver conditions, requiring a combination of clinical assessments, laboratory tests, and imaging studies to provide a comprehensive overview of the liver's health.

Clinical Assessments: Skilled healthcare professionals begin by conducting thorough medical histories and physical examinations. Symptoms, lifestyle factors, and risk factors are carefully considered to guide further diagnostic investigations.

Blood Tests: Liver function tests measure the levels of enzymes, proteins, and other substances in the blood that reflect the health of the liver. Elevated levels of certain enzymes may indicate liver inflammation or damage.

Imaging Studies: Non-invasive techniques such as ultrasound, CT scans, and MRI scans are employed to visualize the liver's structure, identifying abnormalities, tumors, or signs of cirrhosis.

Liver Biopsy: In some cases, a liver biopsy may be recommended to obtain a small tissue sample for microscopic examination. This helps diagnose specific liver conditions and assess the extent of damage or inflammation.

Viral Hepatitis Tests: Blood tests are employed to detect the presence of hepatitis viruses (A, B, C, D, or E) and guide appropriate treatment plans.

The diagnostic process is a collaborative effort between healthcare providers and patients, involving open communication, thorough examination, and a strategic selection of tests to ensure accurate diagnoses. This comprehensive approach allows for the development of tailored treatment plans, emphasizing the importance of early and precise diagnosis in managing liver conditions effectively.

How healthcare professionals diagnose liver diseases

Diagnosing liver diseases requires a systematic and multidisciplinary approach, involving a range of diagnostic tools and expertise from healthcare professionals. The process aims to identify the specific liver condition, assess its severity, and guide appropriate treatment. Here's an overview of how healthcare professionals diagnose liver diseases:

1. Medical History and Physical Examination: Healthcare professionals begin by gathering a detailed medical history, including information about symptoms, lifestyle factors, and risk factors. A thorough physical examination helps identify any visible signs of liver dysfunction.

2. Blood Tests: Liver function tests measure levels of enzymes, proteins, and other substances in the blood that indicate the health of the liver. Elevated levels may suggest liver inflammation, damage, or dysfunction.

3. Imaging Studies: Non-invasive imaging techniques such as ultrasound, CT scans, and MRI scans provide

detailed images of the liver, helping identify structural abnormalities, tumors, or signs of cirrhosis.

4. Liver Biopsy: In some cases, a liver biopsy may be recommended. This involves taking a small tissue sample from the liver for microscopic examination, providing insights into the specific liver condition and the extent of damage or inflammation.

5. Viral Hepatitis Tests: Blood tests can detect the presence of hepatitis viruses (A, B, C, D, or E) and guide appropriate treatment plans.

This collaborative and comprehensive diagnostic process allows healthcare professionals to formulate accurate diagnoses and tailor treatment strategies to the specific needs of individuals with liver diseases. Regular monitoring and follow-up assessments are crucial for ongoing management and care.

The role of imaging studies, blood tests, and liver biopsy

Imaging studies, blood tests, and liver biopsy are integral components of the diagnostic toolkit employed by healthcare professionals to unravel the intricacies of liver diseases, providing valuable insights into the organ's structure, function, and specific conditions.

Imaging Studies: Techniques such as ultrasound, CT scans, and MRI scans offer a non-invasive window into the liver's anatomy. These studies can detect structural abnormalities, assess liver size, identify tumors, and reveal signs of cirrhosis or fatty liver disease. They are crucial for initial assessments and ongoing monitoring.

Blood Tests: Liver function tests measure various substances in the blood, including enzymes and proteins, that reflect the health of the liver. Elevated levels of specific enzymes may indicate liver inflammation or damage. Additionally, viral hepatitis tests help identify the presence of hepatitis viruses, guiding appropriate treatment plans.

Liver Biopsy: In cases requiring more detailed information, a liver biopsy is performed. This involves extracting a small tissue sample from the liver for microscopic examination. It provides a precise diagnosis of specific liver conditions, assesses the degree of inflammation or fibrosis, and guides tailored treatment strategies. While more invasive, a liver biopsy remains a gold standard for certain diagnoses, offering invaluable information for effective disease management.

The synergistic use of imaging studies, blood tests, and liver biopsy enables healthcare professionals to diagnose liver diseases accurately, assess their severity, and devise personalized treatment plans, emphasizing the importance of a multidimensional diagnostic approach in liver healthcare.

CHAPTER SIX

Living with Liver Disease

Living with liver disease presents a unique set of challenges that extend beyond the physical symptoms, encompassing emotional, social, and lifestyle aspects. Coping with a chronic condition requires resilience, adaptability, and a comprehensive approach to well-being.

Physical Challenges: Individuals with liver disease may experience fatigue, pain, nausea, and other symptoms that impact daily life. Managing these symptoms often involves medical interventions, lifestyle modifications, and adherence to treatment plans.

Emotional Well-being: Dealing with a chronic illness can evoke a range of emotions, including anxiety, depression, and stress. Building a support network, including healthcare professionals, friends, and family, is crucial.

Mental health considerations are an integral part of holistic disease management.

Lifestyle Adjustments: Dietary changes, limitations on alcohol consumption, and modifications to daily routines are often necessary. Adopting a liver-friendly lifestyle, including regular exercise and stress management, becomes essential for overall health.

Social Impacts: Liver disease can affect relationships, employment, and social activities. Advocacy and open communication about the condition help reduce stigma and foster understanding among peers and colleagues.

Financial Considerations: The cost of medical care, medications, and potential lifestyle adjustments can pose financial challenges. Seeking support from healthcare providers, social services, and community organizations can alleviate these burdens.

Navigating the complexities of living with liver disease requires a multidimensional approach, emphasizing physical health, emotional well-being, and social support. Education, self-advocacy, and a proactive stance towards healthcare contribute to a better quality of life for individuals facing the realities of liver disease.

Coping with a new diagnosis

Receiving a new diagnosis, particularly for a chronic condition like liver disease, can be emotionally overwhelming and challenging. Coping with a new diagnosis involves a multifaceted approach that addresses the physical, emotional, and practical aspects of the situation.

1. Education and Understanding: Seek information about the diagnosed condition, its causes, symptoms, and treatment options. Understanding the nature of the disease empowers individuals to actively participate in their care.

2. Building a Support System: Reach out to friends, family, and support groups. Sharing the diagnosis with loved ones fosters emotional support, and connecting with others who have experienced similar situations can provide valuable insights and coping strategies.

3. Emotional Well-being: Acknowledge and express your feelings. It's normal to experience a range of emotions, including fear, sadness, or anxiety. Seeking the support of mental health professionals can assist in navigating these emotional challenges.

4. Developing a Treatment Plan: Work closely with healthcare professionals to develop a comprehensive treatment plan. Understand the recommended therapies, medications, and lifestyle modifications necessary for managing the condition.

5. Lifestyle Adjustments: Embrace necessary lifestyle changes, such as dietary modifications, exercise routines, and stress management techniques. These adjustments contribute to overall well-being and enhance the effectiveness of medical interventions.

6. Advocacy and Communication: Be an advocate for your health. Open communication with healthcare providers, asking questions, and actively participating in decision-making empowers individuals to take control of their health journey.

Coping with a new diagnosis is a gradual process that involves adapting to change, seeking support, and actively engaging in one's care. It's essential to prioritize self-care and to recognize that it's okay to seek help during this challenging period.

Lifestyle adjustments and support networks

Lifestyle adjustments and support networks play pivotal roles in the journey of those grappling with a new diagnosis, particularly for conditions like liver disease. These two elements intertwine to create a foundation for holistic well-being.

Lifestyle Adjustments: A new diagnosis often necessitates modifications to daily routines, dietary habits, and overall lifestyle. For liver diseases, these adjustments may involve dietary changes, limiting alcohol consumption, adopting regular exercise, and managing stress. These lifestyle alterations contribute not only to the management of the condition but also to overall health and resilience.

Support Networks: Building a robust support system is crucial for emotional well-being. Friends, family, and support groups provide invaluable encouragement, understanding, and empathy. Sharing experiences with others facing similar challenges fosters a sense of community and reduces feelings of isolation.

The synergy between lifestyle adjustments and support networks creates a framework for coping and thriving. Establishing healthy habits and having a network of people who understand and empathize can significantly improve the quality of life for individuals navigating the complexities of a new diagnosis. It underscores the importance of a comprehensive, multidimensional approach that addresses both the physical and emotional aspects of health.

Mental health considerations

Mental health considerations are integral components of the broader framework for individuals navigating a new diagnosis, especially for conditions like liver disease. The emotional impact of a health challenge can be profound, affecting one's mental well-being in various ways.

1. Emotional Response: A new diagnosis often triggers a spectrum of emotions, including anxiety, fear, sadness, and uncertainty. Acknowledging and processing these feelings is a crucial aspect of mental health management.

2. Coping Strategies: Developing effective coping strategies is essential. This may involve seeking support from mental health professionals, engaging in activities that bring joy and relaxation, and practicing mindfulness or meditation to alleviate stress.

3. Communication: Open and honest communication with loved ones and healthcare providers is vital. Sharing concerns, fears, and questions contributes to a supportive network and fosters understanding of one's mental health needs.

4. Acceptance and Adaptation: Coming to terms with a new diagnosis involves a process of acceptance and adaptation. This mental adjustment allows individuals to embrace their current reality, make necessary lifestyle changes, and develop resilience in the face of challenges.

5. Seeking Professional Help: Recognizing when professional mental health support is needed is a strength. Therapists, counselors, or support groups specializing in health-related issues can provide guidance and tools to navigate the emotional complexities associated with a new diagnosis.

Addressing mental health considerations as an integral part of overall health care enhances the capacity to cope with the challenges that accompany a new diagnosis, contributing to a more balanced and resilient approach to well-being.

CHAPTER SEVEN

Treatment Options

Treatment options for liver diseases are diverse, ranging from lifestyle modifications to medical interventions and, in certain cases, surgical procedures. The choice of treatment depends on the specific liver condition, its severity, and individual health factors.

1. Lifestyle Modifications: For conditions like non-alcoholic fatty liver disease (NAFLD), lifestyle changes play a crucial role. These include adopting a healthy diet, engaging in regular exercise, and managing factors like obesity and diabetes.

2. Medications: Various medications are employed to treat specific liver diseases. Antiviral drugs are used for hepatitis B and C, while medications to manage symptoms, reduce inflammation, or prevent complications are prescribed based on the underlying condition.

3. Hepatic Procedures: In cases of liver cancer or advanced cirrhosis, surgical interventions may be considered. Liver transplant, where a damaged liver is replaced with a healthy one from a donor, is a definitive treatment for end-stage liver disease.

4. Interventional Radiology: Techniques like embolization or ablation may be utilized to treat liver tumors or manage complications associated with cirrhosis.

5. Supportive Care: Palliative care, focusing on symptom management and improving quality of life, is important in advanced stages of liver disease.

The optimal treatment plan is tailored to each individual, considering the specific liver condition, overall health, and personal preferences. Close collaboration between healthcare providers and patients ensures a comprehensive and effective approach to managing liver diseases. Regular monitoring and adjustments to the treatment plan contribute to ongoing care and well-being.

Medications for various liver conditions.

Medications play a crucial role in the management of various liver conditions, addressing symptoms, slowing disease progression, and targeting underlying causes. Here's a brief overview of medications used for specific liver conditions:

1. Antiviral Drugs: For hepatitis B and C, antiviral medications such as interferons, nucleoside analogs, and direct-acting antivirals are employed to inhibit viral replication, reduce liver inflammation, and prevent complications.

2. Immunosuppressants: In autoimmune liver diseases like autoimmune hepatitis or primary biliary cholangitis, immunosuppressive medications such as corticosteroids, azathioprine, or mycophenolate mofetil help modulate the immune response and reduce inflammation.

3. Ursodeoxycholic Acid (UDCA): Used primarily for primary biliary cholangitis, UDCA assists in bile flow, reduces liver inflammation, and slows disease progression.

4. Statins and Fibrates: These medications may be prescribed to manage lipid levels in individuals with non-alcoholic fatty liver disease (NAFLD) or non-alcoholic steatohepatitis (NASH), addressing associated metabolic factors.

5. Symptom Management: Medications such as lactulose and rifaximin are employed to manage symptoms of hepatic encephalopathy, a complication of advanced liver disease.

It's crucial for individuals to adhere to prescribed medication regimens, undergo regular monitoring, and communicate effectively with healthcare providers to optimize treatment outcomes. Each medication serves a specific purpose within the context of the liver condition, emphasizing the importance of personalized treatment plans based on a thorough understanding of the individual's health status.

Surgical interventions

Surgical interventions play a pivotal role in managing various liver conditions, addressing issues ranging from tumors to advanced cirrhosis. These procedures are often employed when other treatment modalities prove insufficient. Here are key surgical interventions for liver-related concerns:

1. Liver Resection: This procedure involves the surgical removal of a portion of the liver affected by tumors, cysts, or other abnormalities. It is commonly used for liver cancer treatment.

2. Liver Transplant: In cases of end-stage liver disease or irreparable liver damage, a liver transplant may be considered. This involves replacing the damaged liver with a healthy organ from a living or deceased donor.

3. Ablation Techniques: Radiofrequency ablation (RFA) or microwave ablation (MWA) can be utilized to treat liver tumors by destroying cancerous cells through heat.

4. Transarterial Chemoembolization (TACE): TACE is employed for liver cancer treatment. It involves injecting chemotherapy drugs directly into the blood vessels supplying the tumor, combined with blocking these vessels to cut off the tumor's blood supply.

5. Shunt Placement: In cases of portal hypertension, a portosystemic shunt may be created surgically to redirect blood flow and reduce pressure in the portal vein, minimizing the risk of bleeding from enlarged vessels.

These surgical interventions, often performed by specialized liver surgeons or hepatobiliary surgeons, contribute significantly to the comprehensive management of liver diseases, providing tailored solutions based on the specific condition and individual health factors.

Liver transplantation

Liver transplantation stands as a definitive and life-saving intervention for individuals facing end-stage liver disease, acute liver failure, or irreparable liver damage. This complex surgical procedure involves replacing a diseased or damaged liver with a healthy liver from either a deceased or living donor.

Deceased Donor Liver Transplants: The most common type, deceased donor liver transplants, involve obtaining a liver from a deceased individual whose organs are donated for transplantation. This requires a well-coordinated process of organ procurement, preservation, and transplantation.

Living Donor Liver Transplants: In cases where a deceased donor liver is not available, living donor liver transplants become an option. A segment of the healthy liver is removed from a living donor, usually a family member or close friend, and transplanted into the recipient. The liver has the remarkable ability to regenerate, allowing both the donor and recipient to eventually have fully functional livers.

Liver transplantation provides a chance for individuals with advanced liver diseases to regain a high quality of life and, in many cases, a complete recovery. Post-transplant care involves lifelong immunosuppressive medications to prevent rejection and close monitoring to ensure the well-being of the recipient. While the procedure carries inherent challenges, advancements in transplant medicine have significantly improved success rates, making liver transplantation a crucial and effective therapeutic option.

CHAPTER EIGHT

Dietary Guidelines for Liver Health

Dietary guidelines for liver health are essential in managing various liver conditions and promoting overall well-being. These guidelines focus on supporting the liver's functions, reducing the risk of liver diseases, and aiding in the recovery process. Here are key recommendations:

1. Balanced Diet: Adopt a well-balanced diet rich in fruits, vegetables, whole grains, and lean proteins. These provide essential nutrients, antioxidants, and fiber, supporting overall health and liver function.

2. Limit Saturated Fats and Sugars: Reduce the intake of saturated fats and sugars, as excessive consumption can contribute to non-alcoholic fatty liver disease (NAFLD). Opt for healthy fats, such as those found in avocados and nuts.

3. Moderate Protein Intake: Ensure a moderate intake of protein, as it is essential for liver health. Sources like fish, poultry, beans, and legumes are preferable.

4. Control Portion Sizes: Be mindful of portion sizes to maintain a healthy weight. Excess weight and obesity are significant risk factors for liver diseases.

5. Hydration: Stay well-hydrated, as water is crucial for the liver's detoxification processes, helping flush out toxins and waste products.

6. Limit Alcohol Consumption: If alcohol is consumed, do so in moderation. Excessive alcohol intake is a major contributor to liver diseases, including alcoholic liver disease.

Individuals with specific liver conditions may require personalized dietary plans, and consultation with a healthcare professional or a registered dietitian is recommended for tailored guidance. Following these dietary guidelines not only supports liver health but also contributes to overall wellness.

Foods beneficial for the liver

Incorporating liver-friendly foods into your diet can contribute to overall liver health and aid in the prevention or management of liver diseases. Here are some foods known for their beneficial effects on the liver:

1. Fruits and Vegetables: Rich in antioxidants, vitamins, and fiber, fruits and vegetables help combat oxidative stress, reduce inflammation, and support liver function. Include a variety of colorful options such as berries, citrus fruits, leafy greens, and cruciferous vegetables.

2. Fatty Fish: Cold-water fatty fish like salmon, mackerel, and trout are abundant in omega-3 fatty acids. These essential fats have anti-inflammatory properties and may help prevent or manage liver diseases.

3. Nuts and Seeds: Almonds, walnuts, flaxseeds, and chia seeds are excellent sources of healthy fats, antioxidants, and fiber. They support overall health and may contribute to liver well-being.

4. Whole Grains: Opt for whole grains like brown rice, quinoa, and oats over refined grains. These provide fiber, vitamins, and minerals, aiding in weight management and reducing the risk of fatty liver disease.

5. Green Tea: Known for its antioxidant and anti-inflammatory properties, green tea has been linked to improved liver function and may help protect against liver diseases.

6. Coffee: Regular, moderate consumption of coffee has been associated with a lower risk of liver diseases, including liver cirrhosis and liver cancer.

Incorporating these foods into a well-balanced diet can play a crucial role in supporting liver health and promoting overall well-being. Always consult with a healthcare professional or a registered dietitian for personalized dietary recommendations, especially if you have existing liver conditions.

Foods to avoid or limit for those with liver disease

Individuals with liver disease benefit from avoiding or limiting certain foods to manage their condition effectively and prevent further complications. Here are foods to be cautious about:

1. High-Sodium Foods: Excessive sodium can contribute to fluid retention and exacerbate conditions like ascites in individuals with liver disease. Limit processed and salty foods, and opt for fresh, whole foods.

2. Sugary Foods and Beverages: High sugar intake can contribute to non-alcoholic fatty liver disease (NAFLD). Limit sugary snacks, desserts, and sweetened beverages to support liver health.

3. Fried and Fatty Foods: Fried and greasy foods are high in unhealthy fats that can worsen conditions like fatty liver disease. Opt for healthier cooking methods like baking, grilling, or steaming.

4. Red and Processed Meats: Red meats and processed meats contain high levels of saturated fats, which can contribute to liver inflammation and damage. Choose lean protein sources like poultry, fish, and plant-based proteins.

5. Alcohol: For individuals with liver disease, alcohol is a significant risk factor. Abstaining from alcohol is crucial to prevent further liver damage and complications.

6. Refined Grains: Foods made with refined grains, such as white bread and white rice, can contribute to insulin resistance and may exacerbate conditions like NAFLD. Choose whole grains for better nutritional value.

Individual dietary needs may vary based on the specific liver condition, so it's essential to consult with healthcare professionals or registered dietitians for personalized dietary guidance tailored to individual health requirements.

CHAPTER NINE

Special Considerations (e.g., Pediatric Liver Diseases, Genetic Conditions)

Special considerations in liver health extend beyond the common adult population and involve unique challenges related to pediatric liver diseases and genetic conditions affecting the liver.

Pediatric Liver Diseases:
Children can experience a range of liver conditions, from congenital disorders like biliary atresia to metabolic diseases. Managing pediatric liver diseases requires a

specialized approach that considers the child's growth, development, and unique physiological needs. Timely diagnosis, nutritional support, and sometimes surgical interventions are critical components of care.

Genetic Conditions:
Several genetic conditions impact the liver, such as hemochromatosis, Wilson's disease, and alpha-1 antitrypsin deficiency. These conditions often necessitate lifelong management, involving dietary modifications, medications, and regular monitoring to prevent complications like cirrhosis or liver failure.

In both pediatric and genetic liver conditions, a multidisciplinary healthcare team, including pediatricians, hepatologists, genetic counselors, and dietitians, collaborates to provide comprehensive care. The focus is not only on managing existing symptoms but also on optimizing long-term liver health and minimizing the impact of these conditions on the overall well-being of affected individuals, whether children or adults. Tailored and patient-centered approaches are paramount in navigating the unique challenges posed by these special considerations in liver health.

Overview of liver diseases in specific populations

Liver diseases manifest differently in specific populations, influenced by factors such as age, gender, ethnicity, and underlying health conditions. Understanding these variations is crucial for targeted prevention, diagnosis, and management. Here's an overview of liver diseases in specific populations:

1. Pediatric Population: Children may face liver diseases ranging from congenital abnormalities like biliary atresia to metabolic disorders. Timely diagnosis and intervention are critical for ensuring proper growth and development.

2. Adults and Elderly: Non-alcoholic fatty liver disease (NAFLD) is increasingly prevalent in adults, often associated with obesity and metabolic syndrome. In the elderly, age-related changes in liver function may influence disease presentation and management.

3. Gender Differences: Certain liver diseases, like autoimmune hepatitis, exhibit gender-specific patterns. Women are more commonly affected, emphasizing the importance of gender-sensitive diagnostic and treatment approaches.

4. Ethnic and Racial Variations: Some liver diseases show variations in prevalence and severity among different ethnic and racial groups. For example, the incidence of chronic hepatitis B is higher in certain Asian populations.

5. Genetic Factors: Hereditary conditions like hemochromatosis and Wilson's disease impact specific populations due to genetic predispositions. Genetic counseling and tailored management are essential in these cases.

A nuanced understanding of how liver diseases affect diverse populations informs targeted healthcare strategies, promoting early detection, personalized treatment plans, and improved outcomes for individuals across various demographic groups.

Unique challenges and considerations

Liver diseases present unique challenges and considerations that span a spectrum of medical, social, and personal dimensions. These factors influence the prevention, diagnosis, and management of liver conditions, shaping the overall healthcare landscape.

1. Stigma and Awareness: Liver diseases, particularly those associated with alcohol or viral infections, often carry a social stigma. Addressing misconceptions and promoting awareness is crucial for early detection and reducing stigma-related barriers to seeking medical care.

2. Co-Existing Conditions: Many individuals with liver diseases may have co-existing conditions such as diabetes, cardiovascular issues, or mental health concerns. Managing these interconnected health aspects requires a holistic and coordinated approach.

3. Limited Treatment Options: Some liver conditions, especially in advanced stages, may have limited treatment options. Liver transplantation, while transformative, poses challenges related to organ availability and post-transplant care.

4. Socioeconomic Factors: Socioeconomic disparities can impact access to healthcare, diagnostic tools, and medications. Addressing these disparities is vital for ensuring equitable care for all individuals, irrespective of their socioeconomic status.

5. Global Impact: Liver diseases have a significant global impact, with variations in prevalence, risk factors, and healthcare infrastructure. International collaboration is essential for addressing these global challenges, sharing best practices, and enhancing treatment accessibility worldwide.

Navigating these unique challenges demands a comprehensive and patient-centered approach, involving healthcare professionals, policymakers, and communities. This approach emphasizes awareness, education, and equitable access to healthcare resources to improve outcomes and quality of life for individuals affected by liver diseases.

CHAPTER TEN

Future Trends and Research

The landscape of liver disease research is continuously evolving, and future trends indicate promising developments that may reshape prevention, diagnosis, and treatment strategies. Here are some key areas of focus in future liver disease research:

1. Precision Medicine: Advances in genomics and personalized medicine are driving research towards tailoring treatments based on an individual's genetic makeup. Precision medicine holds the potential to enhance treatment efficacy and minimize side effects for liver diseases.

2. Non-Invasive Diagnostic Technologies: Developing non-invasive diagnostic tools, such as advanced imaging techniques and blood biomarkers, is a priority. This can revolutionize the early detection of liver diseases, reducing the need for invasive procedures like biopsies.

3. Immunotherapies: Immunotherapy, already a breakthrough in cancer treatment, is gaining attention for its potential in managing autoimmune liver diseases and liver cancers. Research is exploring ways to harness the immune system to target and eliminate diseased cells.

4. Regenerative Medicine: Investigating regenerative approaches, including stem cell therapies and liver tissue engineering, holds promise for repairing or replacing damaged liver tissue, offering novel therapeutic avenues for chronic liver diseases.

As research in these areas progresses, the future of liver disease management appears increasingly dynamic and patient-centric, emphasizing precision, early intervention, and innovative therapeutic modalities. Ongoing collaboration between researchers, healthcare professionals, and technology experts will be essential in realizing these advancements.

Ongoing research in the field of hepatology

Ongoing research in hepatology, the study of the liver and its diseases, encompasses a wide range of investigations aimed at advancing our understanding of liver-related conditions and improving patient outcomes. Some notable areas of ongoing research include:

1. Non-Alcoholic Fatty Liver Disease (NAFLD): Given the rising global prevalence of NAFLD, ongoing research focuses on understanding its underlying mechanisms, identifying biomarkers for early detection, and developing targeted therapies to prevent disease progression.

2. Viral Hepatitis: Ongoing efforts continue to enhance treatments for viral hepatitis, with a focus on developing more effective antiviral drugs, expanding access to treatment, and exploring novel strategies such as combination therapies.

3. Liver Transplantation: Research in liver transplantation aims to optimize organ allocation, improve post-transplant outcomes, and explore alternative therapies to transplantation, such as bioengineered liver tissue and xenotransplantation.

4. Precision Medicine: Advances in genomics are driving research towards precision medicine for liver diseases. Tailoring treatment strategies based on an individual's genetic profile holds promise for more effective and personalized therapies.

5. Immunotherapy: Investigating the role of immunotherapy in liver cancers and autoimmune liver diseases is a growing area of research. Efforts are focused on harnessing the immune system to target and eliminate diseased cells while minimizing collateral damage.

Ongoing research in hepatology reflects a commitment to addressing the evolving challenges posed by liver diseases, paving the way for innovative diagnostics, treatments, and therapeutic approaches that hold the potential to transform patient care.

Emerging treatments and technologies

The field of hepatology is witnessing a surge in emerging treatments and technologies that show promise in transforming the landscape of liver disease management. These advancements span various aspects, from innovative therapies to cutting-edge technologies:

1. Gene Therapies: Gene-based treatments are being explored for liver diseases, offering the potential to correct genetic abnormalities, reduce inflammation, and restore normal liver function. This approach holds particular significance for genetic liver conditions.

2. RNA Therapies: RNA-based therapies, including RNA interference (RNAi) and antisense oligonucleotide therapies, are being investigated for their ability to modulate gene expression and disrupt disease processes. These technologies show potential in treating conditions such as viral hepatitis and genetic liver disorders.

3. Nanotechnology: Nanoparticle-based drug delivery systems are being developed to enhance the targeted delivery of medications to liver cells, maximizing therapeutic efficacy while minimizing side effects.

4. Regenerative Medicine: Advances in regenerative medicine, including stem cell therapies and tissue engineering, offer the possibility of repairing or replacing damaged liver tissue. These approaches are explored for their potential in treating chronic liver diseases and reducing the need for transplantation.

As these emerging treatments and technologies progress from research to clinical applications, they hold the potential to revolutionize the management of liver diseases, providing more targeted, effective, and personalized interventions for patients.

Conclusion

In conclusion, the realm of hepatology, dedicated to understanding and addressing liver diseases, has evolved significantly, offering a nuanced understanding of liver health, diseases, and innovative treatment modalities. The liver, a vital organ with multifaceted functions, is susceptible to various conditions ranging from viral infections to genetic disorders and lifestyle-related diseases.

The comprehensive exploration of liver diseases has revealed the intricate interplay of genetic, environmental, and lifestyle factors. This understanding has paved the way for tailored approaches to prevention, early detection, and management. From lifestyle adjustments and dietary guidelines to cutting-edge treatments such as gene therapies and regenerative medicine, the field continues to expand its arsenal against liver diseases.

The emphasis on precision medicine, incorporating genetic insights and personalized treatment plans, signifies a transformative shift towards more effective and patient-centric care. Ongoing research, fueled by advancements in genomics, artificial intelligence, and regenerative technologies, holds the promise of further breakthroughs in the coming years.

As we navigate the complexities of liver diseases, the integration of emerging technologies, coupled with a holistic understanding of individual needs and socio-cultural contexts, will shape the future of hepatology. With a commitment to awareness, research, and innovation, the medical community is poised to improve outcomes, enhance the quality of life for individuals affected by liver diseases, and ultimately work towards a world where liver health is optimized for everyone.

Recap of key points

In recapitulation, our exploration of liver diseases and hepatology has highlighted several key points:

1. Liver Functions: The liver, a vital organ, performs diverse functions, including detoxification, metabolism, and synthesis of essential proteins, crucial for maintaining overall health.

2. Global Impact: Liver diseases, encompassing a range of conditions from viral hepatitis to non-alcoholic fatty liver disease, have a significant global impact, affecting diverse populations with varying risk factors and prevalence.

3. Types of Liver Diseases: We delved into common liver diseases such as hepatitis (A, B, C, D, E), cirrhosis, non-alcoholic fatty liver disease (NAFLD), and alcoholic liver disease, understanding their causes, progression, and complications.

4. Risk Factors: Lifestyle factors, including diet, alcohol consumption, and viral exposure, contribute to the development of liver diseases. Awareness of these risk factors is essential for prevention.

5. Diagnosis and Treatment: Diagnostic tools, including imaging studies, blood tests, and liver biopsy, aid in the accurate diagnosis of liver conditions. Treatment options vary from lifestyle adjustments and medications to surgical interventions and liver transplantation.

6. Emerging Trends: Future trends in hepatology involve precision medicine, non-invasive diagnostics, immunotherapies, and regenerative medicine, offering innovative approaches to liver disease prevention and management.

Navigating these aspects collectively underscores the importance of holistic, patient-centered care, grounded in awareness, research, and the integration of cutting-edge technologies to enhance liver health globally.

Encouragement for proactive liver health

Encouraging proactive liver health is paramount for preventing liver diseases and promoting overall well-being. Adopting a liver-friendly lifestyle can significantly contribute to the maintenance of this vital organ. Here are some key points to encourage proactive liver health:

1. Balanced Diet: Prioritize a well-balanced diet rich in fruits, vegetables, whole grains, and lean proteins. This provides essential nutrients and antioxidants that support liver function.

2. Moderate Alcohol Consumption: If consuming alcohol, do so in moderation. Excessive alcohol intake is a significant risk factor for liver diseases, including alcoholic liver disease.

3. Regular Exercise: Engage in regular physical activity to maintain a healthy weight and reduce the risk of fatty liver disease. Exercise contributes to overall well-being and supports liver function.

4. Hydration: Stay adequately hydrated. Water aids in the liver's detoxification processes, helping flush out toxins and waste products.

5. Avoid Smoking: Quit smoking or avoid tobacco products. Smoking is linked to various health issues, including liver cancer.

6. Regular Check-ups: Schedule regular health check-ups to monitor liver function and address any concerns promptly. Early detection allows for timely intervention and better outcomes.

7. Vaccinations: Ensure vaccinations for hepatitis, particularly if at a higher risk. Vaccinations are effective preventive measures against hepatitis A and B.

Encouraging these proactive measures empowers individuals to take charge of their liver health, fostering a lifestyle that not only protects the liver but contributes to overall wellness. Cultivating these habits is a powerful investment in long-term health and disease prevention.

www.ingramcontent.com/pod-product-compliance
Lightning Source LLC
Chambersburg PA
CBHW061013260726
48661CB00005B/2176